ABOUT THE AUTHOR

Dr. O'Connor is Director and Professor, Department of Nursing, Western Connecticut State University, Danbury, CT. She was formerly on the faculty of the Department of Nursing Education, Teachers College, Columbia University, New York City. Dr. O'Connor was an associate editor for the *American Journal of Nursing,* and is presently a member of the editorial boards of *The Journal of Nursing Education* and *The Journal of Continuing Education in Nursing,* as well as the *International Nursing Index.* Dr. O'Connor holds a B.S.N. from Cornell University-New York Hospital School of Nursing, an M.A. from New York University, and an Ed.D. from Columbia University.

Andrea B. O'Connor R.N., Ed. D.

Writing For Nursing Publications

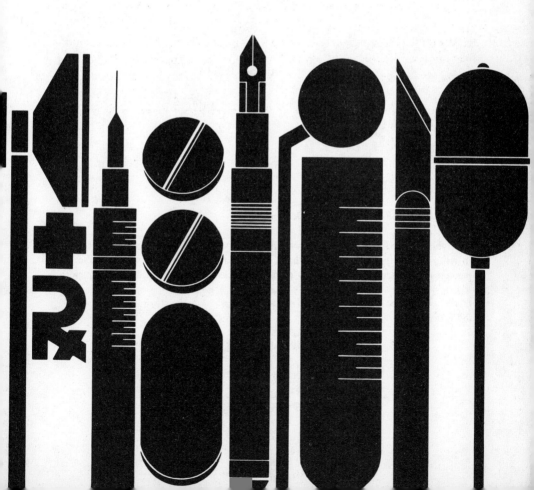

Cover by Anthony Frizano

Library of Congress catalog card number: 81-50881
ISBN Number: 0-913590-77-0

Published in the United States of America by

Slack Incorporated
6900 Grove Road
Thorofare, New Jersey 08086

Writing For Nursing Publications

TABLE OF CONTENTS

With many thanks to TMS, GG, CK, FL, and especially to JOC.

Chapter 1
"Who, Me? Write?"

Yes, you. Write! You have a wealth of experiences, knowledge, expertise, opinions, and discoveries to share with other nurses and health care workers. And one of the best ways of sharing what you have is by writing for nursing publications. Yet you may believe, as many nurses do for one reason or another, that writing for publication is not for you.

"No one would be interested in what I have to say. I don't have a string of degrees after my name."

The authority to expound on some aspect of nursing theory or practice is not tied to educational credentials. You are an authority on whatever it is that you do best in nursing, and you encounter in your daily practice an abundance of raw material that could be the basis of an article. You may not have elaborated a revolutionary theory of nursing science, but in dealing with a specific patient problem you may well have developed a sound approach that would help others in their practice. You may not have done a formal research study, but curiosity about some problem you have noticed in your work may have prompted you to examine that problem in detail, and led you to conclusions that might be useful to others.

Nursing as it is practiced is the foundation for professional knowledge, and is the means by which nursing evolves as a profession. The profession needs its theorists, researchers, educators, and practitioners to help define what nursing is and where it is headed. Only when all nurses share with others what is happening in nursing can the profession grow and develop. You can help in that process, by writing about what you are doing, by sharing information and exploring possibilities with other nurses.

"I haven't got the time. I'm too busy doing nursing to be bothered writing about it."

The very nurses who are advancing the profession through their practice, promoting better patient care, inspiring students and colleagues—in short, the very nurses who are doing nursing—have the most to share through published writing. Writing is, indeed, a time-consuming, lonely, and often frustrating endeavor. It is no easy task to capture in words what is involved in the doing, but those who are at the forefront of nursing have a professional responsibility to write for publication, to look up from their involvement with the doing to recognize that others could benefit from their knowledge and expertise.

But writing is not all giving. Structuring thoughts and delving into unknown aspects of a subject clarify thinking and fill gaps in knowledge. The process of writing helps the writer to critique practice, ask questions, seek relationships, and so enhance future practice.

"I practically flunked English composition. Besides, I don't know all those big fancy words and that technical jargon journals seem to want."

It would be foolish to say that organization of content, sentence construction, spelling, punctuation, and grammar are unimportant. These are essential elements of effective written communication, and can be mastered by anyone. But lofty phrases, flowery prose, and academic "gobbledygook" do not make an article. Rather, pretentious writing often clouds a worthwhile message or serves to disguise disorganization, sloppy thinking, and weak or nonexistent arguments. Clear, precise writing is the best vehicle for communicating ideas, but this is not easily achieved. Thoughtfulness and discipline are required; extensive vocabularies are not.

Furthermore, the communication of knowledge, expertise, observations, and ideas is not a new experience for most nurses. Nurses chart patients' progress, develop care plans, explain procedures to patients and fellow workers, and so on. Each of these activities requires the effective use of words. Writing for publication requires only a few more steps along the same road.

I don't know what I could write about. The idea of writing for publication intrigues me, but how do I get started?"

Write about what you know. What are you most involved with in nursing? What is your area of expertise? What situations do you encounter most often in your practice? Did a recent experience challenge you, make you ask questions, try a new approach? Has a new piece of equipment or a new care technique been introduced into your clinical setting? Do you find yourself particularly concerned about a recurring problem? Have you read an article recently and questioned the author's conclusions or thought that some point had not been covered? Have you been looking for an article on a specific topic and wondered when someone, somewhere, would write it?

Choose a subject that interests you—it might very well interest others. Focus on the familiar, on what you know best. If your clinical expertise is in the care of acutely ill adults, don't attempt to write about the intensive care of neonates or the special problems involved in the long-term care of orthopedic patients, no matter how interested you might be in these subjects. Writing from your own experience enables you to speak authoritatively, tap an extensive store of knowledge, attend to details, and develop your paper in a logical and meaningful manner.

Writing for nursing publications is something you can, and probably should, do. Let your mind wander over potential topics, choose an intriguing one, and start writing!

Chapter 2
Getting Started

Once you have a general idea of what you might want to write about, you will have to make some decisions about your purpose in writing on this particular subject, your potential audience, the general content of your article, and how you might want to approach your subject. These closely related decisions will help you to clarify your thinking and set some guidelines for your writing.

Decisions about the *purpose* of your article answer the question: Why do you want to write on this subject? An article is not a book; all aspects of a subject cannot possibly be covered in the space of a standard-length journal article. Therefore, you must focus your thinking to determine what main point or points you want to get across, what aspects of the subject you wish to stress, what your principal message is. Try to state your purpose in one or two sentences which very specifically describe your central theme. Then keep this theme clearly in mind as your proceed to develop your article.

Decisions about the potential *audience* to whom your article is directed answer the question: For whom are you writing—specialists, nurses in general, nurses in a related field, nursing students, allied health workers? Your potential audience determines how much knowledge you assume the reader has regarding your subject, how generally or specifically you deal with your subject, and eventually, which journals might be most interested in publishing your article. Obviously, decisons about your potential audience are closely related to your stated purpose. The two should be compatible, and together, help determine the content of your article.

Decisions about *content* answer the question: Which aspects of the subject will you cover? Keeping your central purpose in mind, try to list the essential information you will have to present to achieve that purpose. Then, for each item of information you have listed as essential, determine which details promote your purpose and which are extraneous to it, however interesting. Consider your potential audience to determine how much background information you need to provide to ensure that the reader will understand what you are saying, and how deeply you should delve into your subject to meet the reader's need for new information. In attempting to discern your audience's need for information, it is helpful to keep in mind the maxim: Never underestimate the reader's intelligence or overestimate his knowledge. Many novice writers assume that "everyone knows" the basic information underlying the substance of the article. Yet most readers don't know, or don't know in the way that the author plans to use the information in presenting material. Therefore, provide an overview of the basic information you hope to use in developing your article so that the reader can approach the content from your perspective.

Decisions about the *approach* you will use in writing your article answer the question: How do you plan to present the information? What is your organizational scheme? A review of several current nursing magazines will reveal a variety of ways information can be presented. Many subjects can be approached in several different ways; some content must be presented in a specific format; or your potential audience may suggest an approach. In general, the decisions you have made about your purpose, potential audience, and proposed content will help you to determine the approach you will use in writing your article.

Your approach may follow the suggested formats presented below, combine two or more of these formats, or become a totally unique presentation of information. What is essential is the logical organization of your material, an indication of the importance to the reader of the information you are presenting, an explanation of the reasons behind the facts, and an elaboration of the implications of the information for nursing and/or nursing practice.

The **didactic** approach presents information in a straightforward, instructive manner. This approach is applicable to a wide variety of subjects, and is the approach most commonly used in nursing articles. The didactic article presents facts, analyzes them, and usually suggests implications for nursing practice or for situations nurses may encounter as professionals.

The didactic approach is often the best way to review the available information on a timely and important topic, present new information not currently available in the nursing literature, synthesize information from several sources, or draw implications for nursing when this has not been done before. A good didactic article demonstrates the reader's need for knowledge about the subject, explains complex concepts in easy-to-understand language, and explores the ways in which the information presented can be applied in a variety of practice situations. As its worst, the didactic article can easily become a dull review of the literature, a rehash of information readily available in textbooks, or a preachy monologue consisting of a series of "the nurse should . . ."

Clear thinking and a thorough understanding of all aspects of the subject are necessary to write a didactic article. The text should follow some sort of logical format that enables you to present the simpler information first, then move to more complicated material. Unfamiliar terms should be defined and central concepts carefully explained. The tendency for this type of article to be dull can be averted by the use of relevant examples and case histories. Illustrations, such as tables and charts, are often a good way to present complex information (for example, the actions of an enzyme or hormone), lists (for example, drug side effects or interactions), or to relieve a lengthy text.

Clearly, a thorough search of the available literature on the subject you are writing about is necessary. Equally important, however, is the critical thinking you must engage in to develop answers to the question *Why?* in relation to the information you present, and the creativity with which you pose possible applications of the information to nursing practice.

The **case history** approach focuses on a person or group of people during a significant event. The person or people involved, the situation prior to the main event, the actions taken to solve problems, and, occasionally, a follow-up on the person or persons are described. All sorts of patient problems—illness, social, psychological, whatever—can be discussed using this approach, but the case history also can be used to follow a group of nurses, a single nurse, a student, or others through an event.

The case history is particularly suited to the description of an unusual event, the demonstration of effective (or ineffective) nursing care, or the illustration of the application of a concept. A good case history relates theory to practice, guides others to action, and can be a highly readable article, particularly for the reader who has difficulty relating abstract concepts to concrete situations. To accomplish this, the theory must be carefully interwoven into the history, each succcessive aspect of the case being explained in terms of the theory behind the events as they occur or the rationale for actions taken.

Because the case history is based on a real event involving real people, certain elements are essential to its effective presentation. The situation should be clearly described so the reader can understand the problem fully. Provide all the relevant details the reader will need to become involved with the situation. Make the people come alive. What does Mr. H. look like? How is he reacting to the situation? What does he say? Introduce your major "characters" so that the reader can visualize them and react to them.

Finally, deal with what actually happened. Real situations vary greatly from the ideal descriptions usually provided in textbooks: complications occur, mistakes are made, people don't respond as expected. Depicting these real problems helps the reader to equate the events in your article to situations encountered in practice.

The **"how to"** approach is particularly suitable for describing a method of care or other essentially psychomotor activity. If your purpose is to give information about a new or unfamiliar procedure, describe the use of a new or unfamiliar item of equipment, suggest a new way of performing a standard nursing task, broaden the reader's skills, or review a technique in order to correct common errors in practice, the "how to" approach may be ideal.

A good "how to" article captures the reader's attention by indicating why the information being presented is vital. What makes you believe that the reader will encounter the new procedure or equipment in practice? How can patient care be improved by using the technique you are explaining? What is wrong with old way of doing it, and how can your method help? What are the consequences of performing a task incorrectly? Start your article by attempting to convince the reader to read on.

Essentially, the "how to" approach involves the very specific and systematic description of the activity being discussed. Each step in the technique must be carefully analyzed and clearly described. More often than not, illustrations should be used to focus on details or depict actions which are difficult to conceptualize.

It is helpful to keep the question *Why?* in mind as you analyze the activity, and to provide logical answers to that question as you write. Answering the *Why?* avoids a cookbook approach, helps you to convince the reader that your method is best, and enables the reader to retain the information for future use and adapt it to a new situations.

With the **first-person** approach the author relates a personal experience in order to foster reader empathy for others in a similar situation or to prepare the reader to deal with a similar situation in the future. A good first-person article is difficult to write. It is essential to keep your purpose and your audience clearly in mind. Otherwise, this type of article can easily turn into an endless harangue that allows the author to let off steam but generally bores the reader.

The first-person approach can be an excellent way to describe perceptions of the health-care system or of a specific illness state or sensations during a treatment or diagnostic test that would be difficult for the reader to identify without experiencing. Likewise, this approach can be used to describe a problem that the reader is experiencing or may experience and show how that problem may be solved. The first-person article is less appropriate for griping, for presenting information that can easily be obtained in another way, or for relating experiences commonly shared by others.

A first-person article should contain information that is applicable to the reader's situation. These implications for practice should be identified for the reader. For example, information about a patient's perceptions of a diagnostic test can help the reader in planning pre-procedure teaching for such patients. Specify what should be taught. A patient's perceptions of symptoms may suggest nursing actions to relieve discomfort. Describe these approaches. Or the reader may be confronted with a problem similar to the one you have described. Draw conclusions from your experience to help the reader solve the problem and avoid the mistakes you may have made.

The **problem-solving** approach describes the situation in which a nurse (or group of nurses) identifies a problem in clinical practice, education, or administration and sets about to solve it. The reported solution offers to readers a new approach to similar problems they may encounter.

Problem solving is common in nursing practice situations, but because problem solving usually does not utilize a formal research design, many nurses dismiss these activities as relatively unimportant and not worthy of publication. This is unfortunate. The solutions posed may be of immediate value to nurses facing similar situations. Also, the problem-solving article may stimulate formal research studies to verify the utility of the solution.

In developing this type of article, describe the problem clearly, including its origins, if these are known. Indicate why the problem is a problem, if this is not evident. For example, what effects is the problem situation having on patient welfare or convalesence, or on staff morale? Describe previous attempts to solve the problem and why these failed. Then, present your solution. Describe procedures clearly, so that someone else can replicate them. Indicate your rationale for the approach you took, and the steps involved in implementing the new procedure. Finally, describe the outcomes. If possible, document your conclusions by providing "before" and "after" statistics.

If characteristics of your practice situation influence the specifics of the solution your are proposing, indicate this and suggest modifications others may make in adapting the solution to their practice settings. If you encountered problems in implementation, describe these for readers, including steps taken to overcome the problems.

The **research format** is used, obviously, to report study findings. The formal research article follows a specific organizational scheme, providing the reader with a statement of the problem and the purpose and the need for the study; a review of the pertinent literature; hypotheses to be tested; a detailed description of the methods used, including study design, sampling methods, instruments, procedures, data collection, limitations, assumptions, and so on; results, including statistical analyses (often reported in tables); and a discussion of the problems with the study, the implications of the research for practice, and suggestions for further research.

The formal research report requires an attention to details that readers without a research background may find dull. Consequently, important findings may never reach many readers who could apply these findings in their practice. The informal research article enables the researcher to communicate findings to these readers. The informal research article is also useful for reporting the results of an informal study, or of a study in which the sample size was insufficient to draw broad conclusions but results indicated the need for a more extensive study.

The informal research article focuses on the study's implications for practice. The problem and purposes of an need for the study are described, and the theoretical framework of the study, as derived from the literature review, is presented to demonstrate the logic of the study design. Enough information about methods is provided to indicate to whom the study results can be applied and how the study was conducted. The purpose of the informal report is to indicate what was done and why, not to provide information for future replication of the research. The results are reported in terms of trends. Much of the statistical analysis is dropped in favor of interpreting the study results for the reader and outlining the implications of the findings.

The **theoretical** article seeks to communicate a new theory of nursing— a model of nursing practice, a proposal for a change in nursing education or administration on the basis of one or more theoretical constructs, a hypothesis about the relationship between two or more variables—in general, an explanation for or definition of some aspect of nursing or health-care practice. A theoretical article attempts to add to nursing's knowledge base, and requires you to examine your theory rigorously from many sides. In explaining your idea, you will want to provide all of the details necessary to answer the reader's questions about your theory: its logic, its relationship to other theories and to reality, and its potential applications and benefit.

In proposing a new theory, review existing theories or models dealing with the same general problems. Why are those theories insufficient or inappropriate? How does your theory differ from these? Which theories complement your own, or provide a base for your thinking? After you have elaborated your theory in detail, indicate, using examples, how the theory can be applied by identifying situations in which the theory may work and demonstrating how it works. Your theory may or may not be testable; if you believe your theory can be tested, indicate how such research may proceed.

As nursing practice has become more theory based, and theories of nursing have been incorporated into the undergraduate curriculum, a new type of article has appeared in nursing journals. The **theory-testing** article seeks to demonstrate the usefulness of theory as a guide to planning and delivering nursing care or to point out problems with the theory that may lead to its revision. Such articles are essential to the development of meaningful theories of nursing.

A theory-testing article begins with a brief overview of the selected theory, focusing on its essential concepts and their relationships to one another and to various nursing activities. A diagram or other illustration may be used to clarify the conceptual model for readers. Next, case material is introduced in sufficient detail to acquaint the reader with the basic elements of nursing care required. The case may involve an entire patient-care study or a single episode. Cases selected for theory testing usually are straightforward, so that relationship between theory and practice can be drawn clearly.

The case is discussed in a systematic fashion; for example, using the nursing process, applying the theory as a guide to decision making and proposed actions. Then, the theory's strengths and weaknesses are identified, alternative approaches suggested, and, finally, recommendations made for revision of the theory.

Theory testing ideally involves controlled research approaches. Yet, as an applied practice discipline, nursing needs theories that work in real life situations. The theory-testing article provides a means to critique theories in terms of their relevance for practice.

An article dealing with an **issue** attempts to present dispassionately arguments on all sides of the question so that the reader can make an informed judgment regarding a personal stance on the issue. Naturally, the arguments you select and the way in which you present them will refelct your own biases, but the less blatant such biases are, the better chance the article will have of serving its primary purpose.

An issue article requires careful documentation and analysis of prevailing views of the subject. A good issue article presents the issue in context for the reader. Why is this an issue? What historical developments led to the present situation? What aspects of the current scene helped to make this an issue? Why should the reader take a stand on the issue? What effect will a decision, one way or the other, have on the reader's situation? What other issues are related to this one, and how will a decision on this issue alter or affect decisions on related issues?

In summing up your article, you may wish to take a stand on the issue. Your logical analysis of the arguments gives you the authority to do so. Again, however, both the positive and negative aspects of the view you are taking, as well as the positive and negative aspects of the stance you are rejecting, should be presented in summary to give readers an opportunity to form their own opinions.

Closely related to the issue article is the **opinion** article. In stating an opinion, your purpose is to sway others to your point of view. The authority to express an opinion derives from your analysis of pro and con arguments surrounding the issue and your familiarity with and involvement in situations in which the issue arises. You may have a strong opinion about collective bargaining in academia, but if you work in a physician's office there is little chance that you will be intimately acquainted with the ramifications of this problem, and hence your opinion, however solidly rooted in a knowledge of the arguments for and against this issue, will carry less weight than will the opinion of a faculty member or dean. You would, however, be in an excellent position to state your opinion about collective bargaining for physician's assistants.

In stating your opinion you will most likely focus on arguments supportive of your own position and refute opposing contentions. Your own stance concerning the issue will be strengthened, however, by the presentation of relevant arguments against your stance, and their rebuttal.

The **historical survey** approach to a subject is useful for recording the developmental progress of a movement or phenomenon, reporting a current event by placing it in its historical context in order to support its significance, or providing an overview of a movement or phenomenon that has relevance for a present situation.

The historical survey article usually proceeds chronologically; focuses on the situation, the times, and the people involved; develops all three in a logical manner; and relates historical aspects to events occurring today. What events, built on past events, have formed the basis for future developments? What situations at that time caused issues to arise, and what fostered decisions and actions with regard to those issues? Who was involved? What were these people like? What message does history have for decisions regarding today's issues? How did historical events shape the present world? A good historical survey article brings the past alive for the reader, acquaints the reader with personalities, and demonstrates the importance of past events for present-day and future situations.

The decisions you make regarding your purpose, your potential audience, and your proposed content, coupled with your thoughts about possible approaches you may use in developing your article, will provide good direction for your writing. Once you have made these decisions, you are ready to move along in preparing your article for publication.

Chapter 3
Moving Along

Before you actually begin to write your article it is wise to consider potential journals that might be good forums for your work. Dozens of nursing publications are being read by nurses who are eager to learn about the latest developments in nursing care, to hear about new techniques and procedures, to consider the issues related to professional practice today. What's more, the editors of these journals are looking for bright nurse-authors who are willing to contribute to the development of the nursing profession by writing for publication.

The table at the end of this chapter lists a number of nursing and related journals, presented to broaden your horizons concerning the possibilities for publication. The table is by no means all-inclusive. Rather, it lists journals that are representative of the many journals directed to nurses or allied health professionals that may be interested in nurse-authored articles. This list can be a starting point for ideas concerning which journals might appeal to the audience you have in mind and which tend to publish articles similar in content to the one you are planning. After considering possibilities, consult the journals themselves to determine their appropriateness for your purpose and to check on the name of the editor (these change frequently) to whom you will submit your manuscript and for specifications on manuscript preparation. If you cannot locate a copy of the journal, write to the publisher for information on editorial focus and submission guidelines. Both the *International Nursing Index* and the *Cumulative Index to the Nursing and Allied Health Literature* list journals they index, along with the publisher and address.

Keeping your purpose, content, approach, and particularly your audience in mind, select several nursing or related journals you believe might be interested in your article. You will want to consider those magazines that are most likely to reach your potential audience. For example, if you have identifeid an audience of pediatric nurses and your purpose is to describe a specific aspect of the care of infants, you would be wise to consider submitting the manuscript to a specialty journal in this field. If your article concerns a fairly local event, you might want to try your state nurses association's journal. Consider all the possibilities and focus in on three or four likely prospects.

If you are unfamiliar with any of the journals you have selected, or have not read a copy of the magazine for some time, review several back issues to determine if the articles it publishes are similar in content level and approach to the article you are planning to write. Most journals publish a mix of articles to satisfy the varying needs of their heterogeneous audiences, but a highly technical or research-oriented journal is not likely to be interested in an article dealing with a "how to" review of a standard nursing technique. Such an article is more suitable for a general nursing publication or for one directed to allied health workers.

Another point to consider in selecting a possible publisher for your article concerns the number of issues of the journal that appear each year and the number of articles published in each issue. If two journals are comparable in terms of audiences and content level, the more frequently published journal or the one with more articles in a given issue may offer you a better chance of getting your article accepted for publication. Consider new journals too. These tend not to have a backlog of manuscripts and are eager to procure articles for publication. Also, the time lag between acceptance and publication is likely to be shortened.

If your article will require special illustrations (for example, full-color photographs), select a journal that can handle these materials.

Once you have narrowed your choice of magazines, select the one you would most prefer to approach initially and carefully review a good number of past issues (five years back is the furthest you need to go) to determine whether any articles similar to yours have already been published. If so, don't be discouraged. Read these articles carefully. How would your article differ? Do you have a new angle on an old idea? New information to present? An entirely different approach to the content that may prove more helpful to readers? If the published article is very similar to the one you have in mind and was published within the past five years, it is doubtful that the editor will be interested in publishing your manuscript. Try another journal.

Most journals use a refereed system of manuscript review. Copies of the manuscript and a rating sheet are sent to two or more members of the editorial review board. These reviewers are selected for their expertise in the subject matter addressed by the journal. The review process is called a "peer" review because the reviewers generally tend to share the interests and level of expertise of contributing authors, and so are considered to be the best judges of submitted materials. Most journals that use a refereed system conduct "blind" reviews, where the author's name and institutional affiliation are deleted to prevent partiality in manuscript selection.

For those few journals that still process manuscripts internally, usually by nurse-editors, the query letter is a convenient and effective means of establishing contact with the editor and determining the journal's interest in reviewing your manuscript for possible publication.

In the query letter you want to intrigue the editor with your idea for an article, establish your authority to write such an article, and demonstrate your ability to use words and communicate your thoughts. Therefore, you want to be especially careful in writing your query.

In one or two paragraphs, indicate what you plan to write about, including your purpose and a general idea of the content to be covered, how you plan to approach your material, and why this particular article would be of interest or importance to the magazine's audience. You may wish to include an outline of your proposed article on a separate sheet of paper. A query regarding a research study report should also include enough information about the study design and methods for the editor to consider your description of the study from a research perspectives.

If you discovered similar articles in past issues of the journal, specify how your paper would differ from these. If your review of the nursing literature revealed no articles on your subject, mention that fact.

Describe any illustrations you plan to use and indicate how you plan to obtain them. If you will need help with illustrations, ask if such help would be available.

Give enough information about yourself to validate your ability to write on your subject. You want to include your educational background, your work experience, and, in particular, any special experiences you have had that relate to your subject area. If you plan to use a resource person who is an authority in the field, indicate with whom you will be working and why this input will be valuable.

If you are able to do so at this time, estimate the length of your manuscript in double-spaced, typewritten pages and how long it will take you to complete the manuscript.

Write concisely and with precision. Carefully check your spelling and punctuation. As a small sample of your writing, your letter will prompt the editor to speculate about how well written the finished manuscript will be. A good idea presented poorly could well be rejected.

If you know an editor on the staff of the journal you are querying, or to which you wish to send a completed manuscript, by all means send your letter or manuscript to that person. Otherwise, direct your correspondence to the magazine's editor-in-chief, or to the appropriate person, as indicated on the magazine's masthead. If the publisher of the journal you are approaching also publishes other journals, be certain to specify to which journal your correspondence should be delivered.

Refereed journals tend not to process queries, but, instead, request that the manuscript be sent for review. In such instances, submit the manuscript, using a query style letter as the cover letter. This approach will facilitate the editor's direction of the manuscript to appropriate reviewers, and may stimulate sufficient interest by the editor to attend carefully to the fate of your manuscript during the review process.

NURSING AND RELATED JOURNALS

General Nursing Journals

Advances in Nursing Science
American Journal of Nursing
Canadian Nurse
Clinical Nurse Specialist
Computers in Nursing
Journal of Advanced Nursing
Journal of Christian Nursing
Journal of Holistic Nursing
Journal of the National Black Nurses' Association
Journal of Nursing History
Journal of Professional Nursing
Image: Journal of Nursing Scholarship
Imprint
International Nursing Review
Issues: National Council of State Boards of Nursing
Nursing Clinics of North America
Nursing Economics
Nursing
Nursing Forum
Nursing & Health Care
Nursing Outloook
Nursing Papers/Perspectives in Nursing
Nurse Practitioner: American Journal of Primary Health Care
Nursing Life
RN Magazine
Topics in Clinical Nursing

Medical-Surgical

AANA Journal: American Association of Nurse Anesthetists

ANNA Journal: American Nephrology Nurse Association
American Journal of Infection Control
AORN Journal
Canadian Critical Care Nursing Journal
Canadian Operating Room Nursing Journal
Cancer Nursing
Cardiovascular Nursing
Critical Care Quarterly
CONA Journal: Canadian Orthopaedic Nurses' Association
Critical Care Nurse
DCCN: Dimensions of Critical Care Nursing
Diabetes Educator
Dimensions in Oncology Nursing
Focus on Critical Care
Journal of Enterostomal Therapy
Journal of Nephrology Nursing
Journal of Neuroscience Nursing
Journal of Ophthalmic Nursing and Technology
Journal of Post Anesthesia Nursing
JEN: Journal of Emergency Nursing
Heart & Lung: Journal of Critical Care
Infection Control and Hospital Epidemiology
NITA: Journal of the National Intravenous Therapy Association
Oncology Nursing Forum
Ophthalmic Nursing Forum
OR Manager
Orthopaedic Nursing
Perioperative Nursing Quarterly
Plastic Surgical Nursing
Seminars in Oncology Nursing
Today's OR Nurse

Maternal-Child

Birth: Issues in Perinatal Care and Education
Family Planning Perspectives
Health Care for Women International
Issues in Comprehensive Pediatric Nursing
Journal of the Association of Pediatric Oncology Nurses
Journal of Nurse-Midwifery
Journal of Pediatric Nursing: Nursing Care of Children and Families
JOGNN: Journal of Obstetric, Gynecologic, and Neonatal Nursing

Maternal-Child Nursing Journal
MCN: American Journal of Maternal Child Nursing
Neonatal Network: Journal of Neonatal Nursing
Pediatric Nursing
Pediatric Nurse Practitioner

Psychiatric/Mental Health

Canadian Journal of Psychiatric Nursing
Community Mental Health Journal
Issues in Mental Health Nursing
Journal of Psychosocial Nursing and Mental Health Services
Perspectives in Psychiatric Care
Psychiatric Nursing Forum

Community Health

AAOHN Journal: American Association of Occupational Health Nurses
American Journal of Public Health
Caring: National Association for Home Care
Family and Community Health
Health Values: Achieving High Level Wellness
Journal of Community Health Nursing
Journal of School Health
Home Healthcare Nurse
Hospice Journal
Public Health Nursing

Rehabilitation

Journal of Burn Care and Rehabilitation
Rehabilitation Nursing
Sexuality and Disability

Geriatrics

Geriatric Nursing: American Journal of Care for the Aging
Journal of Gerontological Nursing
Long-Term Care Quarterly

Management

Computers in Nursing
Journal of Ambulatory Care Management
Journal of Long-Term Care Administration
Journal of Nursing Administration
Nursing Administration Quarterly
Nursing Management
QRB: Quality Review Bulletin

Education

Computers in Nursing
Evaluation and the Health Professions
Health Education
Health Education Quarterly
Journal of Continuing Education in Nursing
JNE: Journal of Nursing Education
Journal of Nursing Staff Development
Imprint
Mobius: Journal of Continuing Education for Health Science Professionals
Nurse Educator
Patient Education and Counseling

Research

Annual Review of Nursing Research
Advances in Nursing Science
Communicating Nursing Research
Computers in Nursing
Image: Journal of Nursing Scholarship
International Journal of Nursing Studies
International Nursing Review
Nursing Research
Scholarly Inquiry for Nursing Practice
Western Journal of Nursing Research

Allied Health

Journal of Allied Health
Journal of Practical Nursing

Chapter 4
The Nitty Gritty

Organization, clarity, and precision are essential to the effective communication of ideas. An organized article presents thoughts in a logical sequence. Each item of information builds on previously presented material and prepares the reader for the next item. Details surrounding a notion are included at the time the idea is presented. Thoughts flow in an orderly pattern that the reader can follow easily.

Clarity in writing means that each word and phrase is unambiguous. Each sentence is straightforward and to the point: two or more readers will interpret a given statement in the same way and there is no doubt as to the author's meaning.

Precise writing requires accuracy: accuracy in the use of words and in the content presented. Each statement concurs with facts as they are known; each speculation is supported by sound theory. Superfluous words are eliminated.

In developing your original idea for an article you focused on your purpose, your potential audience, and the content you planned to cover and gave some thought to the approach you might use in writing your article. These decisions will provide the framework for your article. As you proceed in preparing your paper, keep this framework clearly in mind and refer to these basic decisions whenever you must answer questions regarding what points to stress and what information to include or eliminate.

As a first step in writing, plan your article from beginning to end. This is best done by making an outline. Start with a general design for organizing the information you intend to include in the article and place each item of information in an appropriate place in the outline. The major headings of the outline will correspond roughly to discrete sections of the completed article; subheadings will become the individual paragraphs. Each section should contain all the points related to the major heading; each subheading or paragraph should identify a single idea or point to be developed.

Fill in the outline from the general to the specific until all the points you wish to include in the final article are placed in their logical order within the overall design. The more detailed your final outline, the easier it will be for you to write your paper.

You want next to identify and fill any informational gaps suggested by your outline. For each item you have entered in the outline, ask those questions a reader might ask concerning that point. What causes this to happen? Who was involved in this event? How was this discovered? Why is this important? Answer each question from your own knowledge or experiential base and/or your review of the pertinent literature. Then sort out which of these answers should be incorporated in the final article in view of your purpose and audience, and which could be ignored on the basis of your assumptions regarding the level of your audience's knowledge or because the details involved in answering the question are irrelevant to your purpose. Fill in the outline with the information you will be using in your paper.

In filling informational gaps do not rely entirely on your memory. Refer to the patient's medical record if you are recording a case history. Ask other people who were involved in his care for their perceptions of his appearance or personality. If you kept a diary or journal during an incident you are reporting, check back to verify the sequence of events and the details surrounding them. If the incident involved a clash with another group (for example, the events involved in successfully negotiating a collective bargaining agreement), attempt to check the opposing group's record of the event to confirm the sequence you have identified and avoid assumptions regarding their position.

When dealing with facts, use recognized, authoritative sources. If differences are noted in two or more sources, determine why these occur and use the source that most fully documents its conclusions. In working with theoretical explanations of phenomena, identify alternate theories and the thinking beyond the theory you find most acceptable.

Your clear thinking and careful preparation to this point have established a firm foundation for your writing. To proceed, you must sit down and write. Despite the availability of a good number of texts on the subject, no one call tell you *how* to write. Guidelines can be offered, but the art of writing can only be mastered by actually writing.

Of course, the basic "tools of the trade"—grammar, punctuation, spelling, word usage—must be applied effectively in writing a scholarly paper. You may find the following basic resource books helpful in dealing with these specific aspects of writing. Three books I believe essential are:
- William Strunk, Jr. and E.B. White. *The Elements of Style* (New York: The Macmillan Company, 1959).

- *Roget's Thesaurus of the English Language in Dictionary Form* (Garden City, New York: Garden City Books, 1936), and
- a good dictionary.

The Elements of Style is a small book that details the essentials of writing in a series of "rules" concerning punctuation, grammar, word usage, and the principles of composition.

Roget's Thesaurus is useful for identifying the word you want when it eludes you, and for identifying synonyms for words you feel are appearing too frequently in the course of your writing. Use the thesaurus to find the *right* word, not a bigger or more "profound" one.

Use the dictionary to verify spellings, to determine whether the word you are using means what you think it means, and to confirm the existence of words. Everyone has unique problems with spelling and proper word usage. Consulting a dictionary is a simple, effective way to overcome these difficulties. When checking on spelling, use the first spelling listed in the dictionary, since this is the most widely accepted form. A dictionary also is useful for determining whether a term such as "part-time" is one word, two words, or hyphenated.

In addition to these basic books, Theodore M. Bernstein's *The Careful Writer: A Modern Guide to English Usage* (New York: Atheneum, 1973) is a delightful guide to the proper use of words, presented in dictionary form. Most common problems of usage and elementary rules of grammar are dealt with in this volume.

A style manual provides rules to live by when you are writing, particularly concerning punctuation and reference citation formats. Because nursing has not yet adopted a single style for professional writing any of the major style manuals can be used. Examples include the American Psychological Association, *Publication Manual* (Washington, D.C.: The Association); William G. Campbell, *Form and Style in Thesis Writing* (Boston: Houghton Mifflin); Kate L. Turabian, *A Manual for Writers of Term Papers, Theses, and Dissertations* (Chicago: University of Chicago Press).

Beyond these, you may want to consult a text on grammar if grammar gives you particular problems. Reading a wide variety of articles and books is also helpful in becoming familiar and comfortable with proper sentence construction.

Computer programs that check spelling, punctuation, and grammar are available for use with word processing programs. These programs scan work in progress to identify errors for subsequent correction. Some programs can be supplemented with a medical terminology dictionary. Certain nursing terms and phrases may or may not be detected as errors by such programs, so it is important to visually scan the final product for errors.

As you write, you will find that it becomes easier and easier to use these "tools of the trade." Refer to your basic resource books as you need them, but don't wait to master all the rules before you begin writing. Write!

Focus on your subject and address the reader. Keep yourself in the background; your personality will emerge in your choice of content and your use of words. This subtle emergence of your personality will constitute your writing style, but style cannot be forced.

Let your words flow naturally. Do not recast sentences in an attempt at sounding erudite. Do not use obscure, flowery words when simple ones will do. Speak directly to the reader, as if he or she were there. One writer may find it best to just write from the top of the head, knowing that initial ramblings will eventually be revised. In this way, patterns of word usage that are most comfortable for the author can emerge. Another may find it helpful to use a tape recorder to capture a natural style. Still another may work from the outline, refining it continuously until the final paper emerges. Try one or several of these approaches and stick with whatever works best and yields a first draft that sounds like you.

Get right to the point. Draw the reader into the article by capturing attention with your first paragraph. This paragraph, the lead, may pose a question, emphasize or illustrate the importance of the subject to the reader, or introduce a problematic situation. An effective lead immediately presents the reader with a reason to read on.

Write in an active voice; use nouns and verbs; cast sentences in a positive form; and use specific, concrete language. Your task is the communication of ideas and information. This is best accomplished by keeping your reader alert and involved in what you are saying, not by lulling the reader to sleep with a plethora of adjectives, adverbs, and circumlocutions.

Write concisely. Eliminate unnecessary words. State each point in the simplest, most direct way possible. Make each word, each sentence, each paragraph count.

Check your first draft against your outline to be certain you have followed your plan of organization, and included all the information you identified as pertinent to your subject. Then, revise and rewrite.

As you revise your paper consider the following questions:

Is the language unambiguous? Could another reader misinterpret my meaning? Rework unclear portions, using different words.

Is the meaning of each sentence clear the first time it is read? Recast clumsy sections, splitting a complicated sentence into two or three sentences.

Are words used accurately in the context in which they appear? Do the words mean what I want to say?

WORDS TO AVOID

Avoid	Use Instead
administer	give
ambulate	walk
approximately	about
ascertain	determine; learn; find out
assist(-ance)	help
the author(s)	I (we)
communicate	talk
considerable proportion of	many
demonstrate, exhibit	show
dependent on	depends
doctor	physician
in excess of	above; more than
facilitate	ease
feel	believe; think
in order to	to
it is apparent, therefore, that	hence
it is possible (probable) that	possibly (probably)
it may well be that	possibly
it seems to the writer	I think
in the present communication	here
individuals	people; persons
the literature	other articles (books)
large proportion of	much
large number of	many
majority of	most
methodology	method
minister to	care for
a number of	several
orientated	oriented
preventative	preventive
prior to	before
a proportion of	some
regime	regimen
reveal	show
small number of	few
sufficient number of	enough
utilize	use
verbalize	talk

Are superfluous words eliminated? Are complex words replaced with simple, straightforward ones?

Does one paragraph flow logically into the next? If not, write a bridging sentence, or use a subheading to signal a shift in content.

Is every fact verified?

Are there any unanswered questions?

Revision is essential to producing a well-written paper. What was said well initially can always be said better. Strive for the clearest, most precise, most concise writing you can achieve. It may take three, four, or more drafts to accomplish, but the final paper will be well worth the effort.

If you are co-authoring the article, each author will be contributing to the development of ideas and the search for additional information. One author, however, usually is selected to do the actual writing. Each author contributes to the critique of each draft, but the final paper should flow smoothly and reflect a single writing style.

Certain precautions and some rules are necessary when presenting technical information.

Drugs: When referring to a drug for the first time, give the generic name followed by the brand name in parentheses. Future references to the drug can be made using either the generic or the brand name. Many journals tend to prefer generic to brand names, but for some medications, such as dioctyl sodium sulfosuccinate (Colace), constant reference to the generic name is cumbersome; combination products, too, are best referred to by brand name. Some drugs are so commonly used and well known that reference to a specific brand name is unnecessary, as with digitoxin or potassium chloride.

It is critically important to be exact in citing drug dosages. The reader is relying on your information and may apply it to practice. Specify the dose, dosage form, route of administration, and frequency of administration. If a range of therapeutic dosages exists, give that range. If the medication is administered in varying doses on the basis of weight, provide this information as well as an illustration of its application. For example, gentamicin sulfate (Garamycin) may be administered to adults with life-threatening infections in dosages up to 5 mg./Kg./day; hence, an adult weighing 60 Kg. (132 lb.) could be given up to 300 mg. of gentamicin per day.

If alternate dosage forms are available, as with penicillin, indicate of which you are speaking. If you are citing an unusual dosage of medication given in a special situation, it is helpful to give the normal dosage range in parentheses. When referring to solutions or ointments, state the strength being used as well as the quantity being administered.

Many journals prefer the metric system for reporting drug dosages as well as for other measurements; some accept the apothecary system. Whichever you use, use it consistently—and accurately.

Laboratory values: Report normal laboratory values in ranges and indicate what the value refers to (for example, mg./100 ml; mEq./liter; mm. Hg; mg./24 hr.). If you are reporting a specific, abnormal value, as in a case history, give the normal range for the parameter being reported if you have not already indicated this; for example, "Mr. G.'s serum potassium was 2.5 mEq./liter (normal: 3.5-5.0 mEq./liter)." Avoid using abbreviations such as *K, Na, Hct,* and so on; write out what is being measured. An exception to this guideline is generally made in the reporting of arterial blood gas values (pCO_2, pO_2, pH).

Abbreviations: When in doubt, write it out. Eliminate all possible sources of ambiguity. A nanogram (ng.) is much different from a milligram (mg.), but the uninformed reader could assume you meant milligram. Write it out. Microgram can be abbreviated μg but, again, can easily be confused with mg. Write it out.

When first referring to an organization, department, or other commonly abbreviated title, write out the full name followed by the abbreviation if you intend to use it repeatedly: American Nurses' Association (ANA), National Labor Relations Act (NLRA).

Gender: Publications differ in their preferences regarding gender specific pronouns. Some use the he/she, his/her format, which may be distracting to readers. Others direct authors to avoid the gender problem entirely by reworking sentences to eliminate pronouns, which is difficult for the author and may result in clumsy writing. Occasionally the problem is solved by a footnote apology indicating the author's use of conventional gender assignment despite awareness that there are men in nursing and women in medicine.

Don't allow the gender problem to interfere with your writing. Use the pronouns that are most comfortable for you and change them during revision if necessary.

As you work on your article, particularly while you are filling informational gaps, you want to think about your eventual need for footnotes, references, and/or a bibliography. Footnotes usually provide information that supplements the main text of the article; references, although they may be printed as footnotes, are usually listed at the end of the article and cite the original sources of materials used in the article; bibliographies are listed at the end of the paper and contain background or supplementary sources used by the author in preparing the article.

In general, references serve to give credit to the original source of a theory or idea, to document the author's use of certain factual data, and to guide the reader to additional informational resources. The majority of articles published in nursing magazines cite references, but a good number of articles do not use or need them.

All quotations should be supported by a reference. You are free to quote up to 150 words of a given work without obtaining permission to do so from the holder of the copyright. However, you want to be conservative in your use of quotations. Your article should represent, for the most part, your own thinking. You proably will want to quote an author whose unique turn of phrase is particularly fitting or whose controversial statement is germane to your article, but, beyond this, paraphrase or summarize the author's work. Quotations involve the reproduction of another's work; that reproduction should be accurate in *every* detail, including punctuation. Recheck every quotation you use to be certain it is exact. And never quote an author out of context. Your use of the quotation should reflect the author's view.

Paraphrasing is the restatement of ideas in another form. However, some writers merely substitute a few words in a statement or reorganize the statement in an effort to bypass the use of a direct quotation or the work involved in truly interpreting the author's work in their own words. A too close adherence to the original text borders on and easily can turn into plagiarism. Restatement, *using your own words,* is an acceptable way of reporting others' works. Such works should always be cite in the references. To claim another's theories or ideas as your own is also plagiarism. The ideas and conclusions of others should be cited in the references. Obviously, such statements as "Jones concluded that . . ." or "Smith believes . . ." require a reference, but general statements ("It is theorized that . . .") also require references.

If you are supporting the description of a phenomenon with an explanation based on a theoretical conclusion, cite the originator of the theory. If you are dealing with obscure or unfamiliar facts, use references. These citations will be very useful to the reader who wishes to pursue your subject in greater depth by consulting supportive sources.

Different resource books may give varying information regarding drug dosages and laboratory values. It is helpful, in these instances, to support your use of specific numbers by citing your source and by using the most authoritative and current source available.

Whenever possible, use original sources. If Davis refers to Adams, Brown, and Conners, read Adams, Brown, and Conners and cite their original works.

You do not need to cite references for your own conclusions, theories, and opinions. Statements of common knowledge or accepted fact, likewise, do not require references. Above all, do not seek out reference sources when they are unnecessary. Allow your statements to stand and be judged on their own merits.

The format or style for references and bibliographies varies. Select the format currently used by the journal to which you plan to submit your article, or the one described in the style manual you are using. In general, references include all the information necessary to enable the reader to easily locate the original work. For articles, give the author(s), title of the article, journal, volume number, inclusive pages, and date of publication; for books, give the author, complete title of the work, place of publication, publisher, and date of publication. References for quotations should include the number of the page containing the quotation. Materials cited as references should have been published. However, unpublished doctoral dissertations and certain mimeographed materials are occasionally used as references. The citation of "personal communications" should be avoided. The titles of journals can be abbreviated using the standard abbreviations listed in the *Index Medicus,* but when in doubt, write it out.

Writing is a highly personal endeavor. You will develop your own method of writing and your own idiosyncracies within that method. Don't allow a conception of what a writer *should* do to act as a block to your own writing. Use whatever crutches you need to accomplish the task.

Recognize blocks to writing and deal with them appropriately. Every writer experiences blocks at some time. One signal is avoidance behaviors, such as a sudden compulsion to clean the house or wax the car. Often it is wisest to give in and satisfy the compulsion in order to remove the block. Creativity involves more than sitting down and writing; sometimes the time spent in physical tasks releases the mind to work with ideas.

Another major block to successful writing is time—finding the stretches of uninterrupted time needed to develop a coherent paper. Writing frequently proceeds in phases: finding the idea, focusing the article, developing the outline, collecting information, writing the paper, revising. Approach the task in its parts to avoid being overwhelmed. When it is time to write, however, set aside the time you need (a weekend, a series of evenings) and permit no one to violate it.

You have worked long and hard to produce a final manuscript that is well written and accurate in every detail. You are ready to prepare your paper for submission.

Prepare your manuscript double-spaced on standard-sized, white, non-erasable, bond paper. A double-spaced manuscript is easier to read than a single-spaced paper. White bond paper avoids the see-through effect produced by the use of onion-skin paper, an effect that is distracting to the reader. Double-spacing also facilitates the editing process, as does the liberal use of wide margins. Editorial changes usually are made directly on the original manuscript before the paper is prepared for the printer. Double-spacing and wide margins provide ample room for such changes. Editorial alterations usually are made in pencil. Erasable paper presents problems to the editor when he changes his mind and tries to restore your original writing after he has changed it. Computer-generated papers are acceptable provided the printer produces a final copy that duplicates well and is easy to read. Some dot matrix printers create hard copies that work well for rough drafts, but strain the eyes. These should be avoided in preparing final copies of the paper for submission.

Submit two copies of the manuscript (or more if the journal requests them) and retain one copy for your own reference. Additional copies of a manuscript are usually requested to facilitate the review process, especially when the manuscript must be sent to several reviewers. Most journals also retain a copy of the manuscript in their files to insure against loss.

Number each page and include your name at the top of each page for ease of identification. (If the journal conducts a blind review, your name should appear on the title page.) Many manuscripts are reviewed, edited, and prepared for the printer at the same time; shuffling of papers can occur.

If the journal requests an abstract of the article, submit this on a separate sheet of paper placed in front of the main text of the article. The abstract should be a short paragraph (about 500 words) outlining the key points you have made in your paper. References, bibliographies, and biographical information should also be submitted on separate sheets. If the article is based on a funded project, be certain to acknowledge the source of the funds, including the grant number.

Many journals have developed standard specifications for the submission of manuscripts. Consult a current issue of the journal for this information or write to the managing editor of the magazine to obtain a copy of these specifications, and follow the instructions exactly.

Proofread the final copy carefully. If errors appear or you wish to make major changes (for example, if a sentence has been dropped, or you are unhappy with the way a sentence reads, or you wish to add information), retype the manuscript. Of course, such changes are easy to make if you have used a word processor to prepare your manuscript. Typographical errors and last-minute, pencilled changes are distracting to the reader. A clean, corrected manuscript indicates that you value your own work. Your aim is to submit an attractive paper that the editor or reviewer can read without difficulty.

Staple or clip the manuscript at the top left-hand corner. Do not bind the manuscript in a fancy folder or encase it in plastic-coated sheets. A simple staple or clip also makes reading and, eventually, editing easier.

Mail your manuscript flat, in a manila envelope. Your cover letter should refer to any previous correspondence you have had concerning the article, request that the manuscript be reviewed for possible publication, and indicate your willingness to make any revisions the editor may identify as necessary to produce a paper acceptable for publication. Be sure to include your current address. Some journals require authors to sign a statement before the manuscript is reviewed conveying copyright ownership to the publisher. Include this statement in your cover letter or on a separate page. Actual transfer of copyright does not occur until the manuscript is published.

When your manuscript arrives at the editor's office it will be reviewed using either of two processes. Internal review by the journal's editorial staff may be accomplished with or without consultation with advisory panel members or content experts. In a peer-review, or refereed process, the journal sends submitted manuscripts to members of its editorial board who are experts in the content areas covered in the journal. In both cases the manuscript is evaluated using specific criteria, and a recommendation to accept, to request a revision or rewrite, or to reject the manuscript is made. Most manuscripts are reviewed by several editors or board members, and the final decision made by the journal's chief editor.

Once you have submitted your manuscript, you will be waiting with bated breath for word regarding its fate. The review and evaluation of manuscripts is a time-consuming process, and may take several months. However, if six months elapse without word, write to the editor. The manuscript may have been lost in the mail or buried under the piles of paper on a busy editor's desk. If you move while your manuscript is still being evaluated, be sure to inform the editor of your change in address so that word of the disposition of your paper can reach you as quickly as possible.

Chapter 5
Illustrations

Illustrations can be used to provide supplementary information, clarify explanations, or strengthen the human interest aspects of a story. All sorts of graphic materials are used to illustrate articles, including tables, charts, graphs, diagrams, drawings, x-ray films, electrocardiographic tracings, and photographs. Not all articles need illustrations, but many can be enhanced by their appropriate use. Therefore, it is a good idea to give some consideration to the possibility of submitting pertinent illustrations with your manuscript.

Each publication has its own requirements for the submission of illustrations and its own limitations on the kind of illustrations it can accept. These requirements and limitations are often determined by the size of the art staff, printer's specifications, the magazine's format, and budget. The general guidelines that follow will help you in deciding which, if any, of the many kinds of illustrations you should consider submitting with your article. But, always check with the magazine's editor for specific directions regarding submission.

Tables and charts are used to report statistical data and to present detailed information in a compact form. Generally speaking, tables and charts should supplement the text, not repeat it. In fact, their use can solve some writing problems. It is distracting for the reader to struggle through cumbersome lists of numbers and facts that have been integrated into the text of the article, and presenting this information in the text can be a difficult task for the writer. These problems can be avoided by pulling such information out of the text and presenting it in a table or chart, where it can be easily digested. Charts also can be used to summarize information presented in the text. Such charts provide the reader with a reference for future use. Consult several back issues of nursing journals for ideas regarding how tables and charts can be organized and what information is best presented using given designs.

You want to be as careful and accurate in constructing your tables or charts as you were in writing your article. Check all of the facts. Attend to every detail.

Organize the information sensibly. Use simple headings to clearly identify what information is being presented in each section of the chart. Your purpose in using a table or chart is to facilitate the reader's understanding of the data presented. The reader should be able to follow the chart with ease, not spend time figuring out how to read it.

Check your chart for internal consistency. Cast statements in a positive form and use the present tense. Each phrase or statement should follow the same format. Use punctuation and abbreviations consistently. If you are tabulating statistical data, add up your numbers and verify the totals you are reporting. If inconsistencies occur due to your methods of data collection or data manipulation, indicate the reason for the discrepancy in a footnote.

Select a title for the table or chart that conveys its contents in as few words as possible. The reader who is skimming the magazine may be drawn to your article because the chart catches the eye and the title suggests the article's worth.

Tables and charts should be prepared on white bond paper for submission. Include your name at the top of each page. Again, use generous margins and double spacing. Check that all the rows line up for ease and accuracy in reading. Number all the tables and charts consecutively, and refer to them in the text of your article. Your reference to the illustration should identify its contents, not repeat them. For example, "Chart I lists the drugs used to treat tuberculosis," or "The results were tabulated (see Table IV)."

Be certain to document the sources of information used in constructing your tables and charts. Obviously, statistical data generated in your own study need not be supported by references. Charts that summarize points documented in the text also require no references. If the information in your chart was drawn from a single source but organized to create the chart, your footnote to the chart should read, "Based on information from . . .," followed by the source, including page numbers. If you worked from existing charts but presented the information in a unique way, your footnote can read, "Adapted from . . . ." Charts and tables copied in whole or part from existing sources must be treated like quotations and their use usually requires the permission of the copyright holder. Publishers usually are willing to grant such permission. Permission is not required for the reproduction of published government statistics and other information in the public domain. If in doubt, however, write for permission.

Write to the publisher, indicating exactly which chart or table you wish to reproduce, why you wish to use it, and the journal to which you are submitting your article. The copyright holder's written permission should accompany any such charts submitted. The credit line should read "Reprinted from . . .," "Source . . .," or "Reprinted [or used] with permission from . . . ." Be certain that your reproduction of the table or chart is accurate in every detail.

Graphs are used to present statistical information in a visually appealing format that enables the reader to grasp numerical relationships and trends at a glance. Trends and relationships between variables are best visualized in a line graph; comparative data can be presented in either line or bar graphs; bar and "pie" graphs can be used to demonstrate ratio relationships.

As with tables and charts, the information presented in graphs should be clear and precise. Labeling should be simple and to the point. Avoid cluttering the graph with miscellaneous information. If you are using a line or bar graph, label the horizontal and vertical axes clearly, and provide sufficient information about interval lengths to ensure accurate interpretation of the data.

Select a title for the graph that indicates its contents. In addition, provide a caption or legend that will guide the reader in interpreting the graph. As with tables and charts, indicate the sources used in constructing the graph.

Graphs should be drawn with India ink on heavy, white paper. Alternatively, computer-generated graphics can be used if they are clear. Lettering should be large enough to remain legible when reduced for publication. Many journals require professional lettering; a few will prepare the graph for you if you provide the basic information to be included.

Number the graphs consecutively and refer to them in your text. Type all the captions and reference information on a separate sheet of paper. Label the back of the graph with your name and the number of the illustration for ease of identification.

Diagrams are used to explain complex concepts visually. Illustrations in this category range in complexity from the use of arrows to connect a sequence of words to elaborate schematic drawings. Again, a review of several nursing journals may suggest ways in which you can use diagrams to present information.

Diagrams cannot substitute for text; rather, they serve to highlight specific relationships and/or sequences described in the article. Your clear, verbal explanations are essential; diagrams will assist the reader in following these explanations and conceptualizing them.

Simple diagrams can be prepared with India ink on heavy, white paper, and should be submitted like graphs. More intricate and very detailed diagrams may require professional preparation. Before going to the time and expense involved in producing a finished diagram, submit a sketch of your idea for the diagram, complete with title, caption, and other identifying information. The journal's editor or art director can then guide you regarding its suitability as illustrative material and provide specifications for its final preparation.

Drawings can be used to provide visual descriptions in place of verbal ones, or simply to decorate an article. Decorative art is the concern of the magazine's art director; the text of your article will suggest aspects to be highlighted in such drawings. Descriptive visuals can either be suggested or submitted by you. Another group of illustrations discussed in this section, and frequently seen in nursing magazines, are sample nursing care plans, assessment guides, and other forms used to record information.

Descriptive drawings save words by showing rather than telling the reader. They serve the same purposes as demonstrations used in teaching. You want to closely coordinate these visuals with your text, so plan ahead for the kinds of drawings you will need. Then, as you explain, for example, a surgical procedure or the use of a piece of equipment, you can refer the reader to the drawing and avoid lengthy verbal descriptions. Although photographs also may be used for this purpose, the schematic representations achieved in simple line drawings may simplify the visual description by eliminating extraneous details and focusing on the most significant aspects of the item or situation. Some articles require a mix of photographs and drawings.

As with diagrams, you may choose to prepare your own simple drawings or submit a sketch that gives a good idea of what you would like in the finished drawing. In any event, label those details of the drawings the reader should note, submit captions on a separate sheet of paper, number the drawings consecutively and indicate their appropriate positions in relation to the text, and supply identifying information.

Sample forms for recording and communicating patient care information, determining optimum staffing patterns, conducting nursing audits, and other record-keeping tasks are frequently used to illustrate articles about new approaches to this whole area of concern. They are descriptive visuals in that the reader can see what the form looks like, saving you the trouble of describing it. This kind of illustration is most helpful and more interesting visually when the form is filled in.

Submit two copies of each form with your article. Provide identifying information on the back of the form. Fill in one copy of the form as it would be used in the situation, using India ink if the information normally would be handwritten. Use common abbreviations if necessary (pt, c̄, PRN,

B.I.D.), but write out unfamiliar abbreviations. If you referred to a specific case or situation in your text, use information related to that case or situation for the form. Again, number the illustrations consecutively and refer to them in your text.

Photographs provide human interest and also can be used as descriptive visuals. If you are writing about people or events, consider using photographs. Photo sequences also can serve to illustrate a "how to" article, demonstrating discrete aspects of a procedure. For the most part, use action photographs. Posed photographs tend to be stilted and dull. Have your subjects engaged in an activity related to your text. Of course, posed photos are necessary for demonstrations.

Each person who appears in the photographs you submit with your article must consent to the use of the photograph. The written consent must clearly indicate your intention to have the photographs published. The journals to which you are submitting your manuscript may provide consent forms if institutional forms are unavailable. Submit all consent forms, including your own if you appear in a photograph, with the illustrations.

Crisp, clear, black and white photographs printed on glossy paper reproduce best for publication. An ideal size is $5'' \times 7''$ or $8'' \times 10''$, but photographs can be enlarged or reduced without difficulty if the details are clear. Most publications cannot use color photographs, and those journals that do print full-color photographs generally confine their use to specific situations where color is necessary to convey information (for example, color distinctions related to the diagnosis of specific diseases or healing processes). Color reproduction is an expensive printing process, and this is the main reason for its restricted use. Color photographs can be printed in black and white, but may lose clarity in the transition. Obtain glossy prints of slides for submission.

Glossy photographs also should be obtained if you intend to use x-ray films to illustrate aspects of your article. If lettering or other marks are necessary, have this done professionally.

Identifying information (name and the number of the picture as cited in the text) should be typed on a label and pasted on the back of the photograph. Avoid writing directly on the photograph since the pressure involved in doing this can distort the quality of the picture. Indicate which edge is the "top" of the photograph, if this is ambiguous. Type the captions for each photograph on a separate sheet of paper, and be certain to identify each person fully.

If at all possible, send two prints of each photograph. Do not mount the pictures on cardboard or paper; removing them later for use could result in tears. Instead, protect your photographs by placing them in a separate manila envelope between sheets of cardboard.

Electrocardiographic tracings and similar recordings present special reproduction problems because they are usually fragile and can be damaged easily. Some publications require the submission of glossy photographs of such tracings. If lettering or other marks, such as arrows, are necessary, have this done professionally, as with x-ray films.

If the journal will accept the original tracing, mount it carefully on heavy cardboard. Paper cement is best for doing this, since mistakes can be corrected and extra paste rubs off without damaging the original art. Submit a longer tracing than might be needed for publication. Protect the tracings with a sheet of heavy tissue paper, and place identifying information on the back of the art, as with photographs. Do not write on the original tracing. Instead, use a photostatic copy to identify the correct position of arrows and other information. Again, number the tracings in sequence and submit captions on a separate sheet of paper.

Accuracy is as essential in illustrations as it is in writing. Examine photographs closely for breaks in technique. Check charts and diagrams for spelling and other errors. Verify all the information you use in preparing your illustrations.

The appropriate use of good illustrations can enhance your article. Plan for them as you develop your manuscript. Discuss your ideas with the magazine's editor. The editor's suggestions can be invaluable in helping you to prepare illustrations to accompany your article.

Chapter 6
And Then . . .

At last, you hear from the editor. The review of your manuscript has resulted in acceptance; or a request for a revision; or a suggestion that you rewrite; or rejection of your manuscript. After your initial elation—or depression—has passed, read the letter carefully.

A letter of acceptance may include a request for additional information or clarification of some point you made in your article. The editor may suggest certain illustrations and ask you to obtain these, or request that you prepare and send finished copies of illustrations you proposed for your article. The letter may also contain some general information about the editing process and an indication of when your article will be published, as well as a request to convey copyright to the publisher if this was not requested previously.

Acknowledge your receipt of the acceptance letter and send the requested information and/or art as quickly as possible. This will facilitate the editing of your paper later. If you have any questions at all about working with the editor to get your manuscript ready for publication, ask these questions now. If your article contains information that may require updating several months from the date of acceptance, alert the editor to this fact and establish a mechanism for altering the manuscript at a later date to include this information.

Then, get ready to wait again. Although a few articles on subjects of extreme importance are published a month or two after acceptance, most authors wait for six months to a year or more before seeing their articles in print. Each issue of a given journal is planned carefully to provide a balance of content for readers. The articles to be included in each issue are selected from a file of accepted articles. Journal editors review more manuscripts than they can accept; they also accept more manuscripts than may be required for a given issue in order to provide a reserve of manuscripts on a variety of subjects to fill issues during bleak months when few acceptable manuscripts are submitted for review. Preparing an article for publication also takes a good bit of time, although this delay varies from magazine to magazine. It often takes a month or more to edit the articles to be included in a given issue. Typesetting, proofreading, and other production activities may add another month to the process. So, be patient. If six months or more elapse, however, with no word from the journal, feel free to inquire about the status of your manuscript. In the meantime, keep the editor informed about your current address. If the content of your article will be outdated rapidly, warn the editor of this possibility at the time the article is accepted, and arrange for the opportunity to update critical facts immediately before publication, or for the return of the manuscript if publication will be delayed too long.

Instead of accepting your paper for publication immediately, the editor may request a revision. Generally, such a request indicates that you have chosen a timely and important subject but that your paper needs more work before it can be published. A revised manuscript usually has a good chance of being accepted for publication.

The editor may ask you for additional information, or suggest a shift in your focus. The paper you submitted may be too lengthy, and require cutting by a half or a third. After your hard work to submit a perfect paper, such a request may seem unreasonable or impossible, but consider the suggestions for revision carefully. The editor's primary concern is the journal's readers and the editor's objective is to satisfy their needs. At the same time, the editor would like to help you to prepare a paper that can be published. The investment of time and effort in suggesting a revision is clear evidence of this. Your purpose in writing is to communicate with the journal's readers. The suggested revision may well be the best way to accomplish your goals.

If you decide to revise, write to the editor indicating your willingness to undertake a revision of your paper. Ask any questions you have about suggestions, and establish a deadline for submitting the revision. Then follow the editor's suggestions exactly and revise the manuscript quickly. If, however, you firmly believe that the suggested revision would distort or destroy the meaning of your paper, you may decide not to revise. Write to the editor, thank him or her for reviewing your paper, give your reasons for not revising, and submit your manuscript elsewhere.

A letter suggesting a rewrite is similar, in some respects, to a request for a revision; you have selected an interesting subject and the editor believes you can discuss that subject, but your submitted manuscript leaves a great deal to be desired. A suggestion that you rewrite is discouraging, but rewriting is worth the effort. Analyze the editor's suggestions. They may be rather global, but probably will indicate the main problem with your manuscript. Be critical with yourself. Is your paper too narrow in focus? Is the subject developed in depth? Do major questions remain unanswered?

Does the writing ramble on and on and fail to arrive at conclusions? Is the approach suitable? Could the information have been presented more clearly, or in a different way? Reconsider your original decisions regarding your purpose, audience, content, and approach. Should these decisions be altered in any way?

After critiquing your paper, start again with a new outline. Rethinking your entire paper may well reveal errors you made in some early stage. If you think a rewrite is possible, write to the editor and indicate your plans for the paper. Ask for any reactions. Then rewrite your paper and submit it again.

For the most part, manuscripts are declined because of duplication of material on file or poor selection of audience or subject area. If you receive a letter declining your manuscript on the basis of duplication, submit the paper elsewhere. Otherwise, rethink your paper from the beginning, as with rewriting. If you believe you can retain the original idea and rework the paper, do so, and submit it to another magazine. If this seems impossible, find another idea and begin again. Many authors find that their first few papers are rejected. Eventually, they hit on the right subject, the right approach, and the right journal—and receive a letter of acceptance instead of a rejection slip. Keep trying! Each new effort brings you closer to producing a manuscript worthy of publication.

Editing and production procedures vary from journal to journal but generally include the following steps.

When your manuscript is finally scheduled for publication in a specific future issue of the magazine, it will be assigned to an editor for copy editing. Copy editing involves correcting punctuation, spelling, and faulty grammar; tightening loose writing or loosening writing that is too terse and tight; retitling, if necessary; inserting sideheads—in essence, refining the paper so that the article conforms to correct English usage and to the style adopted by the magazine. (In this sense, style refers to preferences regarding punctuation, the use of certain abbreviations and symbols, and so on.) Some magazines have their editors confirm facts, check quotations for accuracy, and verify references; other magazines assume that the author has attended to these details. At this time, final plans for illustration are made and any additional information required from the author is noted.

The edited manuscript is then prepared for the printer. A copy may be sent to you with a letter specifying the nature of and reasons for any major changes that were made in the manuscript, requesting additional information required for the article, and asking you to signify your approval of the manuscript as edited. Read the edited copy carefully. Does the copy reflect your thoughts accurately? Is your style intact? Have significant facts been eliminated? The edited version of your article may not conform word for word to the manuscript you submitted and your favorite phrases may be gone; editors try to produce the best possible finished product while retaining the essence and spirit of the original paper. Does the edited copy reflect this?

If significant editorial changes have been made that distort your meaning, indicate this in the margins of the copy. Provide any additional information requested, and update aspects of the article if this is necessary. But don't quibble over insignificant details. The editor has a good feel for proper sentence construction and word usage. Trust these judgments insofar as the changes involved do not alter your meanings. Indicate your approval of the copy as corrected and return it quickly. Some journals do not send edited copy to authors. These journals usually make only minor editorial changes so that the manuscript conforms to the journal's preferred style of punctuation, reference citation, and so forth. If for some reason you wish to review edited copy prior to publication, indicate this at the time the article is accepted.

As the publication date approaches, the whole publication process speeds up from its initial snail's pace. However, your receipt and return of edited copy does not guarantee the article's appearance in a specific issue. Some articles do get "bumped" for one reason or another. The journal probably will notify you just prior to the actual publication date.

Your review of edited copy is usually the last you will see of your manuscript before publication. A few journals send authors galley proofs for review in addition to or instead of edited copy. Read these carefully, and make only those changes that are absolutely necessary. Authors usually are charged for changes made in galley.

The changes you indicate on your copy of the manuscript will be transcribed to the printer's copy and forwarded for typesetting. Galleys are proofread by the editor and then copy is laid out as it will appear on the printed page. At this time, minor changes may be made to fit the article in the space available. Captions for illustrations are written and art work is prepared for the printer. Final proofs of the pages of the issue are read and approved. The issue goes to press—and you are a published author!

And then? Friends and family congratulate you on the appearance of your article. You receive letters from people you haven't heard from in years—and maybe from people you don't even know. Letters to the editor regarding your article may appear in later issues of the journal. Years from now, someone may refer to your work. A good article may prompt requests from editors of other magazines for an article on a similar or related subject. You are free to write for any publication, but you must write a new and different paper.

On occasion, someone may write requesting more information or citing a difference of opinion or questioning a statement you made. The editor may ask you to respond in writing so that your reply can appear in the magazine's letters column. Respond immediately and graciously. Cite additional references in support of your statements, or elaborate on the reasoning behind your opinion. If an error did appear in the article, admit it and supply a correction in your reply.

You may receive numerous requests for reprints of your article. It is your responsibility to respond to such requests. Reprints can usually be purchased in bulk from the publisher. Wholesale photostatic reproduction of the article for distribution is an infringement of copyright (the publisher usually holds the copyright on material printed in the journal) and should be avoided.

And, by all means, write another article. In fact, as soon as your first article is accepted by a nursing journal, you should start planning and writing another article for publication.

Chapter 7
A Final Note

The rights and responsibilities of authors and editors, which have been alluded to in the preceding pages, are summarized and explained below.

Submit your article to only one journal at a time. Much time and effort is expended in reviewing manuscripts for publication. The editor has the right to assume that if your manuscript is accepted for publication it can be published without the risk of losing it to another journal or, worse, finding that the accepted manuscript has just been published in another journal. Some journals require a written statement from the author indicating that the manuscript has not been submitted elsewhere for consideration. Your voluntary statement to this effect can be included in your cover letter at the time you submit the manuscript.

Verify facts and obtain necessary consents. You are responsible for the accuracy of all facts, statements, quotations, and references which appear in your article. While some journals will undertake the checking of particulars, as the author you remain responsible for the article's overall accuracy. This means that you can be held accountable for libelous statements and for plagiarism.

You also are responsible for obtaining releases for the use of photographs, permission to reproduce charts, tables, and other illustrative materials that have been printed elsewhere, and the approval of your article by the institution or organization with which you are associated, if that institution or organization requires such approval.

Meet deadlines. Whether they are set by you or by the editor, be prompt in meeting deadlines for submitting your manuscript, providing additional information or art work, and returning edited copy. Deadlines help you and the editor complete the work necessary to get your article in print. If, for any reason, you think you will have trouble meeting a deadline, inform the editor in advance and estimate when materials might be sent.

Submit to editing. All manuscripts are accepted with the understanding that they are subject to editing. Even the best articles by the most experienced authors are edited. Graciously welcome this assistance in making your article as well written as possible.

The editor's responsibility to you in this regard is to respect your writing style and preserve your meaning and intent. Your name will appear on the article; you must be satisfied with the finished product.

Request return of your manuscript if you are unhappy. If you firmly believe that editing has distorted your meaning, or if there is an unreasonably long delay between acceptance and publication and no word as to when your manuscript will be published, you have the right to request that the manuscript be returned to you. Until it is published, the manuscript remains your property. Upon its return, you are free to submit it elsewhere.

Glossary

Publishing Terms and Proofreaders' Marks

The language of the publishing world can often be puzzling. A few of the terms and abbreviations you are most likely to encounter are defined below, followed by commonly used proofreaders' marks, which may appear on copy sent to you for approval.

Publishing Terms

1. **art:** illustrations.

2. **au:** author.

3. **blurb:** a summary statement of the content of the article, usually appearing on the contents page; written by the editor.

4. **boldface:** type that is darker than usual.

5. **camera-ready art:** illustrations set on an art board and ready to be photographed for engraving or printing.

6. **caps:** capital letters.

7. **copy:** the typewritten manuscript.

8. **crop:** reduce a picture to fit the space available; usually involves eliminating marginal details.

9. **deck:** an introduction to the article, usually printed in larger type than the body of the article; written by the editor.

10. **F.Y.I.:** for your information.

11. **glossy:** a photograph printed on shiny paper.

12. **ital:** italic type.

13. **makeup/layout:** plans for the page as it will be printed; tells the printer how to position text, illustrations, captions, etc.

14. **mechanical:** art board containing all the elements for an illustration (pictures and type), ready to be photographed for engraving or printing.

15. **ms:** manuscript.

16. **on spec:** on speculation: a manuscript submitted without a prior commitment from the editor to publish it.

17. **over the transom:** a manuscript received by the editor without prior notice.

18. **pic:** photograph.

19. **preprint:** same as a reprint, but printed before publication, usually for special release.

20. **query:** a letter from a prospective author to the editor describing the article the author wishes to write.

21. **reprint:** the final article, usually printed on special stock after publication.

22. **sidehead:** two- or three-word line that breaks the text of the article at intervals.

23. **solicited manuscript:** a manuscript requested by the editor.

24. **stock:** the quality and weight of paper used for printing.

25. **tear sheet:** the actual, printed page of an article, but not bound into the magazine (confusing, since no "tearing" is involved).

26. **unsolicited manuscript:** a manuscript submitted by the author on his or her own initiative.

27. **widow:** an incompletely filled line of type.

Proofreaders' Marks

delete ⟋

close up space ⌣

delete letter and close up space ⟋

transpose letters ⟍

transpose words, phrases ⌐‾‾⌐ (tr in margin)

insert letter, word, phrase ⋀

insert space #

paragraph ⌐ or ¶

run in ⟋

period ⊙

comma ⟋

semicolon ⟋

colon ⊙

hyphen ⌒ = ⌒ / ⋀•⋀

one-em dash   M or em

capitalize ≡   (under letter)

lower case (lc may appear in margin) / through letter

let it stand (dotted line is placed under words to be restored)..........
                                    (stet in margin)

italics _____ (ital in margin)

small capital letters ═ (sm. caps in margin)

bold-faced type ᐱᐱᐱᐱᐱ (bf in margin)

WRITING FOR NURSING PUBLICATIONS

Andy's Handy Dandy List of Helpful Hints

semicolons (;)

Semicolons are used in two ways: either as long commas or short periods, in which case the two clauses (phrases) separated by the semicolon should read as complete sentences (have a noun and a verb), or as serial commas when the clauses in series are complex and contain commas:

EXAMPLES: <u>semicolon as a long comma or short period</u>: Accountability can be demonstrated through a number of processes; peer review, nursing audits, continuing education, and certification are some of the means presently available to achieve this end.

<u>semicolons as serial commas:</u>
Accountability can be demonstrated through peer review, where nurses evaluate each other's practices; nursing audits, where outcomes of care are evaluated based on client records; continuing education, and certification, either for practice competence, excellence, or specialization.

commas (,)

Use sparingly to indicate a break in the sentence. If you can make sense of the sentence without the comma it is usually safe to drop it.

colons (:)

Use to introduce a quote or, rarely, a phrase or question. <u>The question is: Do nurses want higher status?</u> Do not use a colon to introduce a series. <u>The options were (1) apples, (2) bananas, (3) pears.</u>

quotation marks ("")	Use sparingly, if at all, around words and phrases, e.g., "reality shock," "future shock," "burn-out" don't require quotation marks. Save quotation marks for real quotes. In punctuating with quotation marks, periods (.), commas (,), question marks (?), and exclamation points (!) all go inside the marks, but for some strange reason semicolons (;) are left out in the cold.
hyphens (-)	Be guided by your dictionary. In general, hypens are going out of style. Hyphens are most often used to form adjectives and adverbs out of two words: self-interested, well-rounded. Hyphens are not used with the -ly form: partially eaten apple.
apostrophe (')	Apostrophes signal ownership and so are used to make nouns possessive. The singular form of the noun is made possessive by adding 's. EXAMPLE: At the heart of these problems lies nursing's ability to survive. The plural form of the noun is made possessive by adding ' following the s. EXAMPLE: Nurses' willingness to unite in solving problems will make all the difference. Possessive pronouns do not take an apostrophe: my, your, his, her, its, our, their. The exception is one. EXAMPLE: One's ability to practice competently demands more than knowledge. The other use of apostrophes is in forming contractions: don't, won't, it's. A major error is with its as a possessive and it's as a contraction. To detect errors read it's as it is and see if the sentence makes sense. All this means that the apostrophe is best dropped with such items as RNs or 1980s unless you are making them possessive, e.g., the RN's right to strike. By the way, American Nurses' Association uses an apostrophe, but the state nurses associations do not.

parentheses ( )	Phrases in parentheses provide additional information. The material in them can be dropped without losing meaning. (If this is not the case, don't use parentheses.) If the phrase in parentheses is imbedded in the sentence (like this one), use a lower case initial letter and punctuate following the parenthesis (see examples in this sentence). If the clause is a complete sentence it requires an initial capital and its own punctuation.
capitalization	Capitalize all proper names (people, places, associations). Do not capitalize concepts, e.g., nursing, health.
e.g. vs i.e.	e.g. translates <u>for example</u>; i.e. translates, <u>that is.</u> Use e.g. if the illustration is one of several possible examples. Use i.e. only if you are interpreting the one possible meaning of the preceding statement (in which case you probably should have said it clearly the first time) or are presenting an exhaustive list of examples.
abbreviations	If in doubt, spell it out. (This applies to shorthand forms of words, too, such as <u>thru</u> for <u>through</u> and <u>2nd</u> for <u>second.</u>) If you will be referring to an organization, for example, throughout your paper, write its name out the first time and indicate the abbreviation you'll be using subsequently by placing it in parentheses. EXAMPLE: American Nurses' Association (ANA). The use of periods with abbreviations is a matter of style. If your style manual gives you no guidance, however, you can drop the periods (e.g., ANA rather than A.N.A.).
plurals/singulars	Plural nouns (nurses, physicians) and compound nouns (the boy and the girl) require the plural form of verbs. Remember that <u>data, criteria,</u> and <u>phenomena</u> are plurals: their singular forms are <u>datum, criterion,</u> and <u>phenomenon.</u>

which, that	If a clause contains information that is essential to making sense of a sentence, use <u>that.</u> Most <u>that</u> clauses do not require commas. If the clause contains supplementary information, which may or may not be of interest to the reader, so that the sentence makes sense without the clause, use <u>which.</u> Most <u>which</u> clauses are contained by commas.
too, to	too = also or overly. EXAMPLES: I like you, too. We have delayed too long.
effect, affect	effect = result (noun) or cause (verb) affect = influence (verb) or personality characteristic (noun, as in "flat affect")
assure, ensure, insure	The dictionary says they're synonyms, but the shades of meaning are as follows: assure = think "reassure" ensure = think "work to bring about" insure = think "guarantee"
imply, infer	imply: message is given tacitly, or in "coded" form; hinting. EXAMPLE: Does your citation of absentee rates imply that I'm out of the office too much? infer: figure out; deduct. EXAMPLE: Can I infer from your citation of absentee rates that you think I'm out of the office too much?
denote, connote	denote = think "means" connote = think "suggests"
since, because	Picky, picky since: from the time that EXAMPLE: Since the onset of renal transplantation, our hospital has performed X such operations. because: as a result of, or due to EXAMPLE: Because it is a well-known center for this procedure.